Dear Cancer: A Love Letter

By Tan'Yah

Copyright © 2019 by Tan'Yah Global Inc.

Email: Tanya.global.inc@gmail.com
Website: tanyaglobal.com

Ordering Information:
Quantity sales. Special discounts are available on quantity purchases by corporations, associations, and others. For details, contact the publisher at the address above.
Orders by U.S. trade bookstores and wholesalers. Please contact Tan'Yah Global Inc or Amazon.com

Printed in the United States of America/Kingston Jamaica

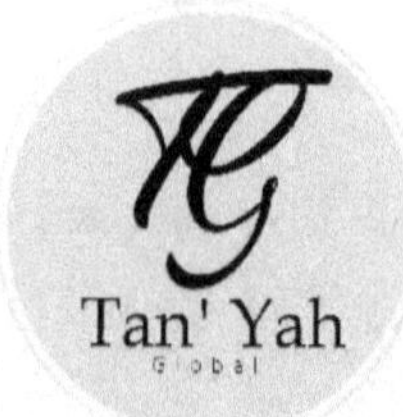

About the Author   4

Foreword   7

Dear Cancer,

'The Unknown One',   10

Dear Cancer,

'Caught in Battle',   17

Dear Cancer,

'Beginning the Healing',   27

Dear Cancer,

'Eye of the Storm',   41

Dear Cancer,

I'm Still Healing,   51

Dear Cancer,

'The people who stayed'   56

Dear Cancer,

'Truth about health'   62

Dear Cancer,

Resources I Used   73

Other Books   74

About the Author

Tan'Yah has been an author, mother, social development expert, researcher, minister of religion, life and health consultant and coach, painter and so much more. It's actually surprising that someone so young could have had the achievements that she has. She however denies any credit and accounts for it as an act of her God – 'Yah' the creator of all things.

Tan'Yah was in the prime of her career as a nationally recognized private consultant and international youth development advocate and specialist in Jamaica when she was diagnosed with triple negative breast cancer. Her international achievements were no small task for a girl from the inner city of Kingston on the small developing island state of Jamaica. She prided herself in very long workdays and was known to integrate her professional and personal life all in one, with her kids regularly seen with her working in the streets across Jamaica.

She was diagnosed with this very aggressive type of breast cancer and was given only two years to live after refusing conventional treatment. While on the journey to recover she did what she did best- learn. As a result, she learned and experienced not just healing but was catapulted into helping others recover their health as well. She became the cancer go-to girl for many and expanded life development to include health and wellness. While she continues in social development through her non-profit ventures, she has committed her life to sharing her experiences and knowledge to others in an effort at changing the world or at least the part she occupies. Her diversity in knowledge puts her in the category of a rare breed of authors and her books cover many different genres.

She came from a very impoverished background and was taught that only hard work would spare her the curse of poverty and this was best achieved through education. And while she started late because of being so poor, she never gave up in her educational pursuits and has achieved an impressive portfolio. She turned down a doctoral scholarship before she started to write this book, as she felt that the most important part of her education now was to dedicate herself to constant learning which has enabled her to become an expert in a new and emerging field. She has melted audiences in international conferences as she helped to shape the language and boundaries of her beloved youth development. And now she melts hearts every time she shares her story of recovery.

An inspiring author who looks back at every experience in her life not with horror but with hope and appreciation that it was all meant for a greater purpose beyond her.

Foreword

Tan'Yah has been down a road that many before her in her own family have gone but were not able to survive to tell the story. Despite being from a hard-natured culture, she has learned to embrace fear not deny it. She has done this restoratively not combatively fueled by what she describes as her love for her God and his purposes for her life. She has learned to dispel taught fear with knowledge. Her journey while not over, has been filled with many hurdles in regaining an optimal state of health, yet she never gives up. I remember her saying for the sake of her kids she knew she couldn't die. As a naturopath I've seen much devastation and Tan'Yah's history positioned her to be another causality, but against many odds she has overcome and sees herself not as a survivor but a conqueror and has grown her body of knowledge from a unique perspective of practicality where she is both teacher healer and student.

And now she can speak up for those that she met that didn't make it and encourage those that can. This book is a heartwarming yet a professional exploration of cancer and what she calls 'the best thing to ever happen to her in life'. Her reference to cancer in the first person is her own skillful way of personalizing this imbalance and identifying it as a part of her.

Keep going Tan'Yah and I hope you inspire others to do as you've done and tell their story.

Dr. Husha Pey

Traditional Chinese Medicine, Naturopath for over 40 years

Dear Cancer,

'The Unknown One',

I have so much to say to *You* about our journey together. I saw you in the distance when you were in relationship with my youngest aunt, who fought being with *You* for years but died a month before *You* were suspected to be on *Your* way to me. Then I saw you again when *You* had relationship with my Dad months before my aunt died. It seems our encounters were many. I also found out when my eldest living uncle by my father died, that *You* and he had been in relationship for many years too. So, you see my first impressions of *You* was not good because those initial introductions were all laced with so much fear of *You,* as attacking and waging war in efforts to kill. I never saw *You* as battling for your own life too. I only saw *You* take over and leave nothing living behind.

Honestly, I like many, feared *You*, because the *You* we've seen or heard of seemed so vicious and so very devasting. When the doctors said *You* had taken over my aunt's life and she would not survive relationship with *You* I was numb, we all were. *You* were this bad dream, or this campaign of horror promoted everywhere. So, when they named *You* and her together forever, we accepted that, and when she in ignorance was told to fight *You* and resist *You*, we supported that too. After all of that, she still died, and we were heart broken. We hated *You*, yet *You* didn't leave, but stayed with my Dad. I felt the fear of *You* from then when I sat with him in the many doctor's offices and even though he was old by their standards, he was still just my Dad and I was not prepared to lose him to *You*. I thought you came to take people, that's what they said, but it just wasn't true was it?

My Dad was so scared he did what they said, even against my advice and that's the effect *You* have on people. The thought of *You*, causes them to ignore rational thinking or any sound advice that goes against the fear of *You*. These by chance encounters forced me to start reading up about *You*. The love for my Dad fueled my hate for *You,* enough to get me started on really exploring the truth of who *You* really were.

I always laughed at the fact that of all things I became in life, a researcher was one of them. I mean I always liked to read and was a quick learner, with a mind overflowing with questions. But come on, me a researcher what a joke, because I was so eccentric and creative. The Creator has a big sense of humor. Who knew I would come to this point of being such a logical strategist with a desire to have evidence to prove the concepts? But in a created plan this was a skill I would need to save and keep my life and allow life to flow from me to the world. And so, *You* became a phenomenon I was desperate to explore, to be able to describe and hopefully conquer. You were still unknown to me personally but through the love for my Dad, relationship with *You* became something I could not ignore.

I looked at the people in oncology related service waiting areas and all I saw was painful devastation, but I was still able to be so thankful for the nurses that were so hopeful, so helpful and so very respectful to them all. I studied how these patients over time changed, their features, even the light of life in their eyes. I saw the lights grow dim and the hope and dignity of their humanness fade from their faces, as their shoulders crouched down, until many of them were seen no more. One day I told my Dad how thankful I was that I was there in treatment with him, as the parent-patient, unlike so many who were there with their children and younger relatives. *You* seemed to love the young. I grew weary not of supporting him but in seeing dismay and death on the faces and in the general deterioration of the bodies who seemed to be waiting to die. My Dad's upbeat approach and his cheery personality kept stirring hope in me and he always nudged me to pray or encourage someone in the waiting area. It was trying to see being with *You* not just a reason to shut down and give up but as an opportunity to reach out to others.

So only a few months later and still going with my Dad to treatment I discovered a lump, from coming in contact with my young son's very sharply shape head back while playing. It pained but at no point did I ever think it was *You* exploring me. I saw the fear on my general practitioner's face the day of my visit, she and I had grown so close sharing baby stories as she admired my young ones. I heard the fear in her voice as she sent me speedily off to do tests. The radiographer's voice was no different and his face couldn't hide his pity for the pretty and smart looking lady he was facing with the results. He'd seen *You* so many times before he was able to say with little doubt *You* and I had started a relationship.

My denial of us being in relationship helped me buy some time to think and I felt that having a lumpectomy would give me me peace for a few months more and then hopefully *You* would be gone.

I opted to be awake during the surgery to have *You* removed and I chose a friend to do it and he was surprisingly hopeful unlike all the other doctors I'd seen up to this point. I figured I would have *You* removed and then tested because I didn't want *You* so close. I chose it that way too, so I could have a moment to breathe with *You* gone.

The urgency in the call to come to the doctor's office told me what I would hear before I heard it and I know as my physician friend gave me the scary news that day that *You* had finally come for me to know *You* were real and we had now entered a relationship together. I was so angry because I didn't think I attracted *You* in any way or at least not intentionally. I smiled, and the doctor thought I was not understanding the severity of the news, but my smile was an acknowledgement that yet again my life was taking a horrible turn but possibly I would make it through as I had so many times before. The doctor took a selfie of us to remind him of the lady who smiled when she was told she had a deadly breast cancer and he promised to pray and keep hope for me alive.

I didn't know *You* and I'm sorry I didn't take the time to find out about *You* before we met. So, I'm writing this book to express my sincere apologies for misunderstanding *You* and treating *You* the way I did in the beginning. I treated you the way I did out of ignorance and fear. I'm also writing for the many friends I've made and lost along the way in hopes that someone will take the time to learn about *You* before ever meeting *You*. I hope writing will help give *You* freedom, so *You* will not seek out more unhealthy relationships and *You* will be at peace. The ignorance about you just fuels more fear of **You.**

I know *You* are scared, and I know *You* are the deep brokenness inside all of us. *You* are the part of me that was over- expose to trauma, harmful pharmaceutical drugs, toxic substances and people, unhealthy lifestyle, self-neglect and malnutrition. I know now *You* were simply bravely crying out for help to save me from myself and a toxic life and environment.

I'm sorry and I hope writing this book will bring *You* greater freedom from within many. And that *You* will experience healing and that it will be your victory. I have learnt that the true therapy we need is not a battle of fighting ourselves to death but loving ourselves to health. So, thanks for giving me the opportunity to share my misunderstanding and our journey together.

Sincerely Tan'Yah

Dear Cancer,

'Caught in Battle',

Again, like many I got sucked into *the world of 'fight against cancer'*. The world that inducts you through fear and ignorance in what allopathic conventional doctors believe to be the only hope. The way my breast was spoken of by the first surgeon and the procedure to cut them off described like they were just two slabs of meat that were only cancerous growths. And then replacing them, being sold to me as such an easy cosmetic job. They weren't treated with any respect, again because **You** were always just being seen as a threat. An imminent threat to my life and survival. **You** were never considered as a part of me that was sick and in need of healing. It shocked, scared and broke me. I know they meant no harm as is in keeping with their code but they like everyone see **You** with such fear, they only enable just that and let's be honest fear can only produce helplessness and hopelessness because it is the absence of faith. One study found that fear and all the negative emotions accompanying it suppresses a person's immune system.

The same system whose failure resulted in *Your* birth and is needed to heal *You*. Now that's irony.

Conventional treatments for cancer follow an international shared protocol of surgery, radiation and chemotherapy and although there have been many other less harmful advances globally with some countries like Latvia changing their protocol to include other less harmful therapies, this is still the general position.

People who are sick generally go to the doctor as an expert in providing diagnosis, treatment and support to recover. But because of how scary *You* are there was just no room for any willingness to consider anything else beyond the recommended protocol for treatment. *You* encouraged me in our relationship to first listen to myself deep within. *You* exposed me to the fact that *You* were me sick and in need of a voice. So, with the support of a naturopath and integrative doctor I was able to learn to listen and trust what **You** would say in response to my biggest question. Why me?

I was the youngest child of a father with a predisposition to reproductive cancers. He had a father, brother and youngest sister dis-eased to those types. But I had three siblings with the same DNA and yet I was the one, why? This was a big question in my diagnosis dilemma I needed answered and despite being told it couldn't be pinpointed *You* said no, and I believed *You*.

The time it takes to heal from decades of mistreatment is long, and so long that conventional medicine says you die first. But the first thing *You* did was force me into myself, so deep that God- Yah had to come and carry me out and take me the rest of the way. So, I knew turmoil better than most, from childhood sexual abuse, abusive relationships, social struggles and mental health issues. But I also knew peace in the storm so, when I decided to chop my two very large breasts off. The same two girls who were often reduced to sources of sexual attraction. For the first time in a very long time I just didn't have-any peace. I don't do much without having a sense of peace and despite my subconscious often takes me into an emotional roller coaster ride first because it was all I knew but, peace always finds me there even if on the exit. So, without peace I refused surgery. And when being issued with a two-year death sentence by the doctor's, my friend peace found its way right back by my side. I think *You* were happy too, because **You** needed peace too and *You* also knew that a mastectomy wouldn't make a difference because *You'd* already made *Your* way to other parts of my body anyway.

The idea of cutting my breasts off wasn't a hard concept for a sexual abuse survivor with huge sexy breast. I always hated them so maybe this was my big break and I would be free without having to make up any big religious excuse to the world as to why they were no more. But without peace this couldn't happen and my hate and resentment for my breast also surfaced as one of the first noticeable emotional enabler of why *You* came. So, I not only made a choice about treatment, but I made a choice about seeking forgiveness for myself from myself and desiring to love the very part of me that was being my pronouncement of death in two years. And what followed was a lot of hugging and I love you-ing to these girls to get them whole and replace with belonginess and appreciation. Yes, cells have memory and so how you feel about pats of your body can make them imbalance and now I'm so thankful for them and I try to learn as much as I can to keep them healthy. This includes lymphatic breast massages, no more tight underwire bras, extra iodide with iodine, less bra wearing and regular chlorophyll with grapefruit seed extract, exercise and jumping around. Yup the girls deserve all my love…they've been through a lot.

Who would have thought such a powerful revelation could come from such a painful decision to get out of the expected normal line. I had been a rebel all my life but finally being a rebel would work in my favor and help save my life.

So, peace came back when I chucked out conventional treatment as an option for me, but *You* were also very much still there too. I still didn't fully realize yet that *You* weren't a foe but a part of me crying out for help for and from me. The pressures of choosing conventional medicine cannot be denied and the exclusion that comes when you refuse it is even scarier than being sick because, you know you're alone for sure. And the search for an undeservingly called quack to help guide us through the unknown is equally hard.

I had grown up with severe respiratory and immune system challenges when I began to be exposed to vaccinations as a very young child. This led to over exposure to antibiotics and removal of parts of my lymphatic drainage system (tonsils, adenoids). I also was a last unexpected child with a fussy appetite which led to poor eating habits and ultimately adult malnutrition, despite I was at my heaviest weight in the advance stages of our relationship. I was usually thin and struggled to maintain the much-loved Jamaican sexy fat. Fat or overweight is never a sign of health which has been a longstanding misconception especially among individuals with smaller body types in many cultures globally. I was also successful professionally with impossible work hours, had insomnia from childhood and ate out most days in poisonous Styrofoam containers and toted my cellular phone in my brassiere quite often. So, one thing is for sure *You* were definitely not uninvited, you were actually prepared for from childhood It didn't help I struggled with trauma, depression and a whole lot of resentment and bitterness. Hence, the question shouldn't have been why me but how come not sooner?

So conventional medicine says fight *You* as an uninvited savage guest. But I learnt that I cannot fight *You* because if I am successful in such a battle, I might kill *You* who is a malfunctioning me leaving the rest of me vulnerable to follow *You* to the grave. So, there is no battle there is only a need to love myself whole and recover my health. In the beginning nobody wants to say thanks to *You* because they fear you might like it and come back, but *You* only came out of a need to be free from physical, emotional, spiritual and environmental poison and pain. Because genetic cancers account for only about five to ten percent of cancers globally, it is then necessary for people to be more responsible and proactive in educating themselves about how to reduce their risk and live healthier lives. Because you play a big role if not the biggest in determining if you will ever have cancer.

The first step then for me was choosing to find a way to heal that I first could believe in wholeheartedly or as near to that as is possible which would enable me maintaining peace. I had to investigate the conventional treatment protocol that was being recommended to me and thankfully social media makes it more than possible to access information and credible data at that. I know people who have done alternative, conventional and integrative. Every person is different and so we must explore what could work best for us or what we can commit our faith and subsequently be dedicated to. Every type and stage of cancer also responds to different treatments in varying ways. Also, all treatment must be holistic whether conventional or non-conventional because each individual is a person with a real life and history before and beyond the dis-ease.

For example, different blood types have different levels of vulnerability to dis-ease and subsequent recovery. So, as an A positive I learned I was already more likely to develop cancer because I was prone to having a depleted immune system more easily that other blood types. This made my survival more unlikely. So even if I had chosen conventional the impact on my immune system by chemotherapy and radiation and surgery would be too great for me to recover from without an immune system therapy. And even doing alternative still left my immune system in a state of vulnerability that required a therapy that could reboot it. Ozone and melatonin therapy finally worked but my body again didn't respond quickly like others and required an intense program and lifestyle to see the recovery of my immune system. I remember always praying for the wisdom Yah to function with my immune system even before I learned this very important lesson on blood types. So, you see my whole man did know what was always needed but I reiterate I was never to taught to listen and let the whole man speak.

You taught me that *You* didn't come overnight and that although unrecognized *You* existed in the shadows of my body until long before *You* were forced to scream and to let me know *Your* pain. When I conceded to *Your* presence and I took the time to listen, *You* told me our story and how *You* came to be. Then you started to show me how *You* had been trying to get my attention when *You* weren't strong enough to speak. **You** caused itching in my breast with heat, lumpiness and even discoloration. But I just never knew I should listen. You couldn't survive in so much oxygen, so I became short winded and tired all the time and *You* craved sugar, so I started to and had many allergies, yeast infections and colds. These along with the many systemic challenges that were going detected but unconnected, like urinary tract infections, indigestion, chronic fatigue, muscle cramp and for a short while just before diagnosis excessively heavy menstrual periods. *You* showed me that *You* were honestly trying to alert me, but my hostile busy life never gave me a chance to see. *You* also showed me how we were never taught to give our physical body a voice and the time to listen when it speaks.

So, thanks for helping me understand how *You* came to be and trusting my whole self to embrace the peace I needed to decide, how I was going to reclaim my health and truly get us healed.

Appreciatively Tan'Yah

Dear Cancer,

'Beginning the Healing',

The decision to do alternative therapies was not the hardest part of recovering my health. After making that decision I then had to maneuver through the overwhelming information that existed first about cancer and then the different genres of naturopathy by whatever name; un-conventional, naturopathic, alternative, natural, holistic, traditional Chinese, Ayurveda or integrative. I had to understand energy medicine, homeopathy, reflexology, herbology or botanical, nutritional, traditional, psychological and so much more. I read more than maybe two dozen articles daily while I was reading a half a dozen books at a time. I started with diet, herbs and reflexology which was good because toxicity was my most urgent issue to address and that was through intense detox. Cutting sugar, integrating whole foods and healthy fats was essential in what I now call a crisis management response (CPR).

Living on an island and a developing nation was now a blessing for a development specialist who was usually the one articulating the negative challenges faced by the country. Access to food endemic to the needs of my racial body type brought joy from the ease of access and the childhood torture of having to be hauled around by my mother as to help with the bags was now a priceless skill I needed to heal with life giving whole foods.

My beloved herbs that often made me gag came with side effects that I needed like sweating, frequent urination, bowel movements, calmness and sometimes appetite loss or gain. Side effects now seem a strange concept in healing because had it not been for this sleepiness, I don't think I could have survived the psychological shifts my life took during this process. Thank Yah I kept falling asleep every five to ten minutes, it was a needed escape from reality and the projecting fear of others.

Reflexology and meridian body massages also really helped my body cope with recovery while helping in removing imbalances of energy all over. These often occurred as part of the healing process as well as initial imbalances that help cause dis-ease.

The body as a whole should be prepared for the many processes of detoxification, nutritional adjustments, rest and rebounding that will be necessary in recovery health. It is good to ease into a treatment plan if you have that option when your dis-ease isn't life threateningly urgent. I obviously didn't have that option with an aggressive fast-growing cancer which was unlikely to respond to much of the convention protocol. So, your mental strength has to be on 'fleek' as the young people would say because everything will usually be very rapid. Your mind will have to be convinced and constantly affirm to yourself that you are healing and you that you will live even if many parts of your life are dying.

I dropped pounds from these initial treatments like ice cream melting in the hot sun and nobody told me until much later that healing sometimes would feel and look like sickness and even death. I was an insomniac for decades so when I began to heal, I began to rest. I would be talking and would fall asleep every five to ten minutes. I could hardly work and when I did, I couldn't manage artificial air or light. This would make me nauseous and foggy. So, in one training I asked them if they would mind me opening the windows and doors to enjoy the beautiful sunlight and fresh breeze of Kingston Jamaica while I struggled to keep my focus and ability to stay alert.

I was eventually almost one hundred pounds coming down from one hundred and sixty and so my physical changes were quite obvious to the world who like small children said the no so smartest things most of the time. My mind had to ignore the ignorant. I also had to ignore how I looked and smacked my emotions every now and again when they reacted to the sight of me in the mirror or walking pass a window at the mall. I had to remind myself that emotions weren't meant to inhabit me but were to help me experience the world outside of me. So, I would just let them express themselves and continue on. They were no longer welcomed as visitors inside my soul no matter how pleasant. I had learnt that they were temperamental and fast changing hence unreliable and so not dependable and beneficial in my recovery.

In this leg of the process you're still solidifying your faith that you are going to live no matter what and that what you're doing will eventually work. The mind has been proven in many researches even by very conventional medical institutions like the Mayo Clinic to be a powerful tool in healing and recovery. So many people utilize meditation and other mental practices focused on helping a person to gain control of their mind in order to better direct their thoughts. So, when the body goes hay wire and looks like its nearer to death than life you have to be convinced yourself that you are on the right track and while you listen closely for your body to give you hints that you're actually healing. For me no matter what, I had a facial glow, disappearing wrinkles and beautiful radiant skin. I also could no matter how weak walk for miles. Logically people who are dying can't do that or don't look that way for prolonged periods of time, so I would look in the mirror and console myself.

Natural therapies produce some visible short-term signs of effectiveness but will need long term application to bring more wholesome healing. So mental strength is needed to sustain faith and commitment. This can be enabled by a positive successful naturopathic practitioner with experience in dealing with severe illness and faith-filled family and friends no matter how few. Kick the nay-sayers out. Respect their views because its often out of love and misguided knowledge but, it is not what someone recovering their health needs. Later you can reconnect when you become the evidence, they'll be more willing to accept other options then.

I've had some friends die in recovery because they just didn't have the mental strength to continue recovering health in the body and the systems affected even after *You* had healed. Because not only does cancer come from deficiencies in the body but it also causes deficiencies that will need to be addressed and healed. The acceptance of your life as it has become is necessary and finding stories of people who were reduced to nothing short of needing resurrection helps to bring real hope. I found the story of a lady with the same cancer, who chose the same path, who had her breasts deflated and body reduced to skin and bones but over time the breast were re-inflated, and the body filled back up. This gave me hope that after *You* and I became one in recovering health we would regain our beauty. I also liked the new skinny version of me because it made me look much younger, so I was in no rush to refill. I also no longer had a husband anymore to be turned off by no breast or anything else for that matter so, I had time and the peace to heal.

A leading oncologist I visited once said she had never seen anyone heal from cancer with natural treatments, but I heard a year later she had since changed her tune. I told her healing is hard for us Jamaicans because it requires healing mentally and emotionally and those were areas that many don't want to explore. We bury the past down deep, and we certainly don't know how to deal with it and so all those harmful emotions and experiences lay buried in our autonomic nervous system reducing the efficacy of our immune and other life systems, because remember everything is connected.

Jamaicans are a people taught to be hard, strong and survive no matter what. Survival is counterproductive to conquering. You can survive something but not conquer it and then you will not be empowered and there's a chance it may come back. This dis-ease requires us to conquer or overcome all the root challenges that led to its existence in the first place. This means we have to be willing to learn and be empowered from the process of healing and recovery making us a light to others coming behind on the same path.

So, there has to be a willingness to be honest and open to keep exposing those wounds while we heal because this is all a process. I was never someone that was willing to be openly vulnerable. I would talk about challenges always from a place of strength but never saw expressing vulnerability as anything but being weak. My physical impairment became so severe I had to learn to be honest about my inability to function at times and ask for help. A big part of this was sharing with those around me how I felt emotionally and physically, in other words being vulnerable so I could receive the support I needed to recover. This was not weakness but true strength another life lessons *You* taught.

 Research showed that most people with breast cancer had faced some traumatic event with a spouse or child. So, treatment must apply the physical tools I've discussed to address imbalances in the body, while we pay special attention in addressing mental and emotional as well as spiritual imbalances in what I call a wholeness approach. I like the Hebrew word for wholeness which means peace and also nothing missing, and nothing broken. To me this defines health and wellness 'Nothing missing, and nothing broken'.

While all these holistic recovery processes are underway, separation as a process and action must also begin. This will be physical for some of our more toxic relationships which will involve drastic separation from many toxic habits and then it will be a separation to within oneself, so we can get to think and engage with the concepts of life and death and other more sensitive issues that others might not understand or appreciate. This act of separation is hard for spouse, children and close friends to understand but it's an act of reclaiming independence. Because, becoming physically in need from dis-ease can rob a person of their dignity and the autonomy which essentially is what really makes us human. I depended on people to drive me around sometimes or stay with me at home to help with the kids and so when I got weaker and my parents encouraged me to move back home, I refused because I needed the separation to heal mentally and emotionally and I needed the freedom to experiment with treatments and develop new routines without judgment or pressure.

This time away while for some will just be a quieting and more internal introspection, it facilitates the rediscovery of self. It's like being introduced to yourself as you have been and who you are becoming, because let's face it, *You* make people different. Nobody is ever the same again and sometimes spouses and close family and friends find that hard to accept because, they want the old you back. But some much of what made you you, also made you sick, so that person should and may never come back. But with the right support this new version could be pretty great. I like living simple and I always have. So, I like the new stress free me who backs toxic people and situations off and is learning to be content. That's me, thankful and trying to remain humble in all things and that may not be what others want but it is who I need to be.

Healing is a process of recovering one's health and so the beginning can seem pretty shocking but, if you keep going and trust your body to not heal itself to death, you'll get there. This process is multifaceted and can only be successful with your commitment to its processes. It took decades to destroy the body for many of us, so we are not going to regain complete recovery of our health in days, weeks, months or even years. Many processes are involved and how the play out in each person is different.

One of the main intensive healing processes

that must be enabled is that of cleaning the body, which includes multiple detoxes of varying types. These have many side effects and some not so great but over time they flush out bacteria, parasites, worms, toxic substances including heavy metals even tumors and other cellular debris. They also help to relieve overload from the liver, gall bladder, kidney and other waste management glands and organs.

Another necessary cleaning process is that of mental and emotional cleaning and rebuilding that can be supported with prayer, mediation, therapy, socializing and even laughing and sleep. I had to take high doses of melatonin until my body created a sleep cycle and if I don't get enough sleep now in a very short time, I feel my body speaking and acting up with all kinds of little issues. I also am learning to laugh and be happy so my body can release the necessary chemicals for health and healing. You see it all comes together

Also, there is the need for physical exercise, sweating, water, sunlight and other tools to support detoxification and physical maintenance while you heal. This takes different forms as the body builds up its strength, but muscles and joints cannot be allowed to get lazy and cease up although healing requires a lot of rest. Research has shown that different blood types require different levels of exercise and so while I'll walk long distances and weight train, intense exercise like aerobics could prove counterproductive to me as an A positive blood type. Physical activity helps the lymphatic system that doesn't have a pump to drain and it also helps the immune system in rebooting.

While the cleaning takes place the process of boosting the immune system through nutrition, herbs, supplements and other treatments has to be in full speed mode, as it is not only involved in this clean or detoxification but is needed to guard and protect while all of this happens. A myriad of nutritional deficiencies of vitamins, minerals and amino acids exist in people who develop cancer and other debilitating illnesses. So, we have to understand that to heal we must not only fill in the gaps but put our body in a state of reserve. At one point I was taking at least 50 nutritional supplements and herbs two to three times daily.

Lastly, there is also the stage of repairing the systems of the body affected by dis-ease like respiratory which includes getting clean air, repairing the liver through herbs and supplements like Milk thistle, stomach and digestive disorders which require enzymes and probiotics and certain diets. So, most dis-eases start in the gut digestive health is key in recovering health and being healed.

So, the processes of recovery are many and unique to each person but while you are being guided by practitioners you must become your greatest expert and listen to your body, so you can ensure effectiveness in healing processes. There are many instances of my doctors recommending something I already discovered for myself or that my body led me through desire to, for example sunlight and exercise.

There were months I just craved being in the sun a lot and walking. Although I generally felt weak and lethargic, I was able to walk many miles in the sun very easily. This was strange because usually the sun felt extremely hot and often felt like it was piercing my skin and would burn me leaving sun burns. But this was no longer the case at all.

I remember it disturbed my father so much when I parked my car and took the bus into the city then walked for miles around running errands or just for the fun of it. He felt that people would think I had lost it and was having some kind of mental breakdown. I didn't care and often laughed and just kept walking. I later discovered the relationship to Vitamin D deficiency and cancer and growing tumors. Yup! I'll stay crazy and just keep walking and soaking up that sunlight. Especially now that I don't burn so easily anymore. The greatest part of getting through the beginning is taking control because live or die the responsibility is yours.

Hey, you, I thank you for forcing me to take control of my life and health. I am so grateful for the encouragement no matter how painful, to face the many toxic situations that faced me and decide to choose life. I learned from you to be consistent in my actions no matter what I saw, and that true freedom will only come if I persevere and believe. I most definitely realize nobody can ever want me to live more than myself and that I must become my own health expert, coach and doctor if my health is to be fully restored and sustained. *You've* changed the way I see myself and others forever and I will never be the same just a better version of me.

Eternally Grateful Tan'Yah

Dear Cancer,

'Eye of the Storm',

So, I continued on my journey and some parts were very secret until lately. One day I was looking at my body in the mirror. I cringed at how much weight I had lost while being contradictorily thankful at the same time. As I inspected me, I realized all the lymph nodes in the network across my upper chest were swollen. I'd learned enough about *You* to know what that meant.

The words of one of the leading Caribbean Oncologist who used alternative treatments as palliative for conventional treatment side effect rings in the ears of my mind. She said nobody she knows has ever healed from using alternative medicine and that many people came back to her after the cancer had spread to other parts of the body like the lymph nodes. Yup, metastasis, well what do I do now right? I heard *You* whisper, we keep going. I was sad at the thought of metastasis, but I really wasn't scared anymore. *You* scared me scare-less. I was faced with the thought of who they said *You* are every second of every minute, of every day and I had become tired of being scared I just had no fear left. I was left empty with faith. It was just like fear emptied me of fear.

So, my sister and I were in a category four hurricane trapped in our Dad's van and as the eye of the storm started the van began to sway from side to side. I looked at my father in the eye of the storm on the porch and I saw his horror, his fear and I knew we were in grave danger. But my Dad swallowed his fear, put his own life at risk to get to us while literally blowing in the wind and he backed that van up into safety. I saw that same fear and horror again in my Dad's eyes as he looked at me facing *You*. I knew I was in the eye of the storm. I was at the point that I was either going to live or die. So, I did a few things.

Learned as much as I could about cancer, health and wellness. Reading journals articles, research, blogs every day.

Got help in making and sticking to my treatment plan. Ask family, friends and people who had done it or believed it could be done to help.

I used the tools of my faith; prayer, fasting, scriptures. Hope keeps the faith to live alive.

Made sure I had herbs that were helping me cope mentally and emotionally. Don't deny how scary it is and use healthy tools to maintain a good mood. Good mood chemicals also help the body to heal.

Surrounded myself with a small circle of people who believed with me. Again, not just faith but faith in action from others helps to keep you here and wanting to stay here.

Made plans. Having a future to live for helps. Hope by every means is essential to fuel faith in the process because the product may not always look so positive.

I loved hard every day and stayed in the now. Nothing beats love. It's like a medicine all on its own.

I didn't deny how I felt physically, emotionally, mentally or financially. Sometimes I felt like I was dying, and I had to say so and get support in whatever way I needed.

Designed a daily routine at every stage. We are indiscipline by nature so to keep on track you have to stick to a routine

There were days I felt like I was going to die. Nevertheless, I knew I was going to live but I felt like death. People around you don't want to hear that especially because you've never died before, but it helps to give a range to how badly you are feeling. My parents hated to hear that the most, but I had to voice that in my healing. I had to be brave enough to face my condition because healing doesn't always feel or look good.

Denial of truth is never a positive thing. As a Christian I was taught to deny sickness and reject symptoms in an effort to stand in my faith about divine health. But healing taught me the opposite. Facing what is, is very necessary in changing or in my case healing and we all know change is a natural part of living. Faith for me says this is my reality and that sickness has gotten a head start for a myriad of reasons and for my faith to catch up I must keep walking in truth.

There was a time in my healing where I would be filled with gas and I felt like the gas was pushing all the oxygen and energy out of my body. I was weak and would ask people to rub my body in order to expel this gas which made me feel better. I had to, for that season accept that belching and farting was what I had to do to live and so I grew out of being ashamed. I use this gross reality because it was mine and accepting and treating with that helped me deal with the side effects of recovering my health. I had to explain to those around me with the visible scary expression of death how I felt, and it help convey the message that I needed sincere help and extreme support to get me through.

As you heal from debilitating and life-threatening dis-ease you will have to face the side effects of not just treatment but also of lifestyle change. My husband left, and it was necessary due to the toxicity of our relationship together. But it was a fourteen-year friendship and an eight-year marriage, so we had a connection. As our relationship split so did our souls and things that had become a part of me were no more. My body that was given a voice now began to sing quite loudly the emotional effects. My progress seemed to turn into regression overnight and I grew even weaker with signs of heart distress. I kept to the list I shared above, and I rode out the eye of the storm. I could smell death as a result of that separation. I could see it and my kids felt it too, as a dreadful fear came into our home. But I kept to the plan, and three months later my body finally started to breathe again. Sometimes you just have to batten down and weather the storm. I listened to my body in that time. When it said it needed sunlight or it needed exercise, or it needed to sweat or sleep. I followed its instruction because it was suffering the most from the trauma. In those times lymphatic massages help to carry me and help energy flow. So, I incorporated whatever I needed to my treatment plan to get me through. Later I've learnt that scientific studies verify my body's instruction of Vitamin D deficiency, muscle weakening, blocked sweat gland and so much more being linked to cancer and my symptoms.

You can't do this however if you or someone supporting you is not reading and growing in knowledge and so I reiterate the point that you must become your own health expert and be able to respond to your changing situation. There were many times I had learnt what to do before even my doctors figured it out. That's the power of the body's voice and the willingness to learn.

Over time the frequency of my healing crises subsided, and I began to maintain more consistent levels of energy and mental focus. The storm was passing, and the radiance of my face was proof. I still used that today to gage my health and respond to my physical needs. There is a song that says the storm won't last always and its true but the secret to riding out the eye is to stay committed and focused to your plan no matter what the human senses say. A plan must be holistic because dis-ease isn't one dimensional. A good plan considers the many facets of your physical, emotional, mental, spiritual, relational and even financial life. Let's face it money answers many things and it took resources in most cases to be unwell and it will take much to recover.

The main challenge I had wasn't getting **You** healed. To be honest that happened quicker than I expected. Let's face it, my body was barely habitable for me, so *You* had to get well to live there. But after all I did, I just wasn't getting my energy back. My body wasn't taking that deep breath. I looked great even twenty years younger, but I was still weak and just not myself. I met a friend who saw very deep within me and recommended I go see and integrative doctor. He was not like any oncologist I had ever met, and he recommended and treated me with ozone intravenously. I didn't get the big burst of life many reported but after three months of diet and complementing coffee enemas I finally started to breathe. My Immune System finally took its first big breath back to life.

Every individual heals differently and healing really doesn't always feel good but one of my Docs always said, 'you'll never heal yourself to death' and I had to hold on to that many times. One thing is for certain our Immune system must reboot no matter how or what enables it. For healing to be sustained it must be charged back to optimal function and every now and again what ever worked must be done to maintain its health.

This is where the science of blood types again is very relevant. Because diet, exercise and lifestyle requirements are different for people of varying blood types its something we must study and incorporate in order to maintain this health we have recovered. Again, this is a change of lifestyle for life not just until you recover and then return to be a dump for toxicity. Remember a dump will always just be a receptacle for garbage and even if you see a plant spring up its still not a farm, just a dump.

I remember on one of my approximately 120-kilometer drives to Ozone therapy I began to cry and ask God-Yah why this all had to be so hard. Each time that needle was stuck into my vein (twice weekly for 12 weeks) I cringed but kept smiling. I remember Him answering me and all my tears dried up and sunshine filled my dark soul. He told me that I was chosen to be His testimony on the earth, and that I truly have become from this journey. I faced all this in order to help others facing *You* too and deter many from ever bringing *You* there. I walked it, to strip fear of **You** from our eyes, so we can see health and healing for what it is - a choice. I'm His testimony.

So, thanks *You* for helping me learn the power of sticking to a plan even in the face of death. This lesson has become very useful in my everyday life since then.

Fondly Tan'Yah

Dear Cancer,

I'm Still Healing,

My business partner asked me to do something the other day and I was reluctant. I had just moved and was trying to adjust as well as just taking in the peace and stability of the moment. So, my partner exclaimed that I was living like someone on vacation and not someone growing a business. I was annoyed but thankful. Why? Because, I'm still healing, and I don't want to live the way I did before. I want to work smart not hard and I definitely want every day to be a vacation.

I've downsized life not just because healing took all the money that life didn't. But I also did it because it gives me greater peace. When you face death as many conquerors do achievements and accolades just don't fill you up the way they did before. The people that you thought were friends who didn't even send a card in all the time of recovery now fade in importance. The profession you invested so much time and resources in no longer seems so important. Death recalibrated me. It set me on a path of priorities of living a full life simply. So, what remains to some is what seems to be a shadow of who I was. But who

I am is free to live healthy and embrace truth as my sustaining treatment for life.

My body has been cleaned and as it gets rebuilt over this next decade, it is now very reactive. So, when I return to eating certain foods or certain poor sleeping or emotional toxicity, I have almost immediate reactions. For example, when I started eating chicken again, I immediately became tired all the time and my weight increased rapidly. I tested it and several times I got the same results, so I had to decide to just shelf that for a lifetime.

I'm still healing or rather we are still healing, and the triggers identified are important to maintain and sustain my health and wellness. I discovered through naturopathic assessments that I had high heavy metal toxicity possibly activated and exacerbated by immunizations, eating from microwaved containers, healthcare products and kitchen utensils like non-stick pots. So, I have to reduce exposure to heavy metals by excluding many products from my life but also by keep detoxing occasionally with charcoal and chlorophyll as well as my beloved coffee enemas.

Another trigger I identified was a limitedly functioning gall bladder that led to many bouts of irritable bowel syndrome in the past with fainting and bitter vomiting. So now I keep up with foods that support bile production and keep up with my liver and gall bladder cleanse a couple times a year or when I break off from diet too far and too long. You might wonder why someone with such a serious history would creep sometimes. Well, it was a part of me for most of my life and so quite often my subconscious tries to pull me back. I have be very careful with the friends I hang out with, or even new friends who may not appreciate my lifestyle because, I was an emotional eater and so can be easily influenced back on the wrong road.

I was a workaholic. My professional and voluntary service life brought me the greatest achievement and high levels of satisfaction and so quite easily I get swept up in doing and I have had to repeatedly step back from my professional life. I have even had to be extreme and move away to a very rural low-key area, where I am forced to enjoy the birds and the sunrise and sunset. The truth is this was the life I've always wanted and was working so hard to retire and have. Who knew with a change in mentality I could have it now? I have to encourage myself to slow down and maintain mental and emotional peace, joy and love.

That's super hard for someone hardwired on stress with serotonin levels through the roof. So, I go to bed early do what I love but in moderation and regularly assess my state of mind and being. It is really hard but when I've ventured far out from this norm, I've had irregularities in my body and health that can lead me right back to **You** screaming my name and crying out for help.

Thank you *You* for reminding me ever so often that you like health, and don't want to return to the way we were. Thank you for teaching my body to be vocal and to become a real advocate for its own wellness. A friend said to me one day that for someone who practices healthy living how come I get so easily imbalanced. I reminded that person that I'm still healing and that - my temple (how I now see my body) is clean so if I pollute it there is an immediate reaction to remove any attempt at pollution and defend itself against whatever it perceives as a possible attack. My kids are the same way the minute they binge at school or out with friends we know because all kinds of ailments begin to show up. This is not sickness its wellness defense and that is just how it should be.

Thank you *You*

Dear Cancer,

'The people who stayed'

Don't get upset or even bitter over the friends or family that can't come with you on a ride like this. Let's be honest we wouldn't either, if we had a choice. I was in a very bad marriage and it couldn't withstand the terror of who we thought *You* were, so it left us even further apart, with a lot of toxicity which meant separation was our only remedy. I think the pain of seeing me or even the thought of me dying was a hard thing to bare and my then husband couldn't handle it at all. During my healing crisis friends stayed away because I looked deathly ill and quite honestly felt like it. I remember one evening I saw the fright in my mothers' eyes, and it scared me so bad. She was on a plane in a couple of weeks because she later explained that she knew she would be no good to me for a while. She had to take a break and regroup. Remember she had a husband in radiotherapy and her youngest child with a death sentence. Was I upset? Nope, I was too weak? Did I finally feel some type of way about it? Nope, because she stood by me more than I could imagine when she got back.

She believed with me while respecting my independence. That's an important thing for someone recovering to feel like they're not living in the third person and that they still have a say in their health journey.

My Dad kept strong while being weak himself and despite his concerns about naturopathy when his body broke down from radiation treatment, he had no choice but to join me and is well even as I type. He prayed many times I know that if one of us had to go it would best be him. I saw it in his eyes, but we are still here together, and we have a bond together that nobody can imagine. Again, Thank You. My father did ozone therapy, detoxes, supplements coffee enemas and herbal teas and a radical change in diet which he struggles to keep and uses his seniority as a weapon in his indiscipline (LOL).

My siblings and their spouses and children have been a fortified city to this day. They've all changed their lives to ensure that family gatherings or visits are healthy and that they are proactive in their own health and wellness. They've respected my choices despite being scared and they've helped financially with loans that they didn't care if I paid back although I have. They've spent the night with me, prayed for me and even been my daily company and clown buddies. They've become best friends and I've learnt to appreciate them in so many ways. To think I use to find family back then boring and spend time and resources in the many friends that dwindled down during this journey.

My daughter was just five and my baby two and my eldest son eighteen when I was diagnosed. Unfortunately, it didn't remain hidden like I wanted it to. And with the other issues of chaos in the house, they were stretched. But while the eldest couldn't speak because he had more untrue knowledge of *You* the little ones didn't and treated me with unconditional love with hugs, kisses, sleeping together, daily prayers and laying on of their little hands. They would constantly remind me that I wasn't going to die and when I couldn't even bathe myself my daughter helped me, and she grew to understand how important it was to rub me and is my personal masseuse to this day. The eldest learned to be independent and stand up for himself because I just wasn't able to anymore because of my physical condition. But they gave me a reason to stick around every second of every minute of every day.

They have had to heal too over time because they have suffered the trauma of perception of **You** and the hardship that comes from their main caregiver not being able to provide for them the way they were used to. But they are kids that have responded to the call of health and they remind me of my needs in keeping healthy.

Family is more than a social concept to me anymore. It's my base and where the core of love resides. I enjoy their company and can share my vulnerabilities because a trust for truth has been established as our family's norm and they still have moments of worry, but I do too for them, because I understand now how to spot imbalance long before it becomes dis-ease. We trust truth now.

Cancer You've changed me and I'm sure it is for the better. I'm not who I was nor am I who I'll be, I don't even hold on so tightly to what makes me, me anymore. And I'm taking the time every day to get to know me and not the reflection of society that I called me.

The few friends that stayed were a blessing and all played a role some would come by regularly for laughs, others would play scientist and want a full explanation of the treatments and their facts and follow-up tests. Others would send money and love and even take the kids out. *You* brought them closer and exposed the beauty of their being to me and that was some of the best medicine I got.

I got so busy doing life that I forgot how to live it and although I had great friends, I didn't have much time for friendship but *You* helped to bring me back to the center and the core of life and the people who we share it with and the need to keep knowing them. It's as if we get to know someone and we think that's all to know so the intensity dies down, but I've learned you can always know me and I'm always knowing others as we keep evolving.

And that's what keeps *Us* free!

My Family and Friend Thanks You

Dear Cancer,

'Truth about health'

We have been taught by modern medicine that colds, diarrhea and allergic reactions just to name a few for example are sickness or symptoms of illness but in truth they are not. They are often the body's natural response to germs, bacteria, virus and signs of imbalance or deficiency in organs and systems. If the body goes through irregular temperature shifts or the lungs or respiratory area become inflamed, mucus and fever is produced as fighting mechanism, but we unfortunately suppress instead of listening to the body and letting things ride a bit and help the body to do its job. Medicine in the West has taken away the body's natural defense mechanism because suppress everything. We have a pain and take a painkiller, so we never learn the why to the pain and the truth to what as to be done. So people think I'm crazy because I let the pain be and pinpoint his genesis, then I respond and it may be something simple while it may be life threatening but, I wouldn't know if I didn't learn to stop, listen, wait and then respond if a response was even necessary because the symptom could very well be the response.

The body is a very complex organism that has been created to function and heal itself and so a healthy person will have cancer cells but will be able to regulate their eventual death if the immune system health is functioning well. We must choose to educate ourselves beyond the knowledge we have been given in the West so we can optimize the body's abilities. And believe me this body has some real superpowers when it comes to healing.

Another truth we must be aware of is that all parts of our self is connected to our health; mental, emotional, physical, spiritual and social. So. we must strive to maintain balance in all of these areas. So, we have people who exercise regularly and are physically fit but are overworked and unhappy and suddenly drop dead one day from a heart attack. When the autopsy is done no cause can be found for the attack. A person who ascribes to naturopathy may deduce he died of a broken heart from stress and no real love connections. A story that inspired me from my favorite book next to bible Radical Remission, was about a Japanese man who had worked sixteen hours a day and now with cancer metastasis all over his body and was given three months to live. He realized very early that his life lacked love and he had lost all real intimate relationship with his family because of his demanding work life. He'd just lost touch which his reality. As he allowed his body to speak and desire clean water and air and love from reconnecting to playing music and his family in less than two years he was in total remission. The final part of that was when he traveled to Great Britain for a couple of weeks. People there hugged him and expressed love a lot. Guess what? That final Cat Scan finally showed no more cancer. It had all gone from him by becoming whole again. We can't ignore the interconnectivity and the need to nourish each part with what it needs. Did you ever notice that when you cry from deep within mucus runs from your body and when you laugh real hard you cough up a lot of mucus? Because grief creeps into the lung and the only way to get sadness out is to express it through tears and laughter. And the mucus being release is a sign of that expression of grief being released. Don't take my word for it, try it.

I realize from my interactions with many women with breast cancer and hysterectomies that we have something in common women who try to thug life out. We are supposed to be strong and try not to display weakness through crying a lot because we've been taught that this being emotionally weakness. Well you do the Math. One study said people who cry a lot are less sick. Hmmm I wonder! Hence, I'm playing catch up with my tears and learning to cry, bawl even.

Another truth about health is you are its master. You can work hard all your life so you can spend it on recovering your health later or you can spend it on living now and not in need of much healthcare later. In Europe they take longer lunchbreaks, maternity and vacation leave and need significantly less sick leave. Why? Because, they understand that the biggest investment you can make in life is supposed to be in you and quality time living. We are taught to educate ourselves for the first twenty years then work hard for the following forty years so we can retire and then enjoy the last twenty something years. You do the Math. Does that make any sense, because if you do like I was you won't have ten good years left when you retire? Your body will be so broken you'll spend every cent of your pension trying to recover your health. Your doctor isn't an expert on you, you are. You know what you need when you need it, but you have to listen learn to quiet yourself and listen to the various parts of your body listen for sensations, heat or cold spots, pain, tension or even tingling. Let your appetite speak and let you know when you are low on certain vitamins, potassium from a banana or vitamin C from citrus or some warmth in the reproductive system from some soup or tea. Give your body a voice and listen. Let's face it doctors are people like everyone else, but the reality is they make money off you being sick consciously or not it really doesn't suite them if everyone is well and so you need to question their knowledge of you and begin to make decisions for yourself.

Statistics say by 2030 as much as one in three persons and in North America it could be as much as one in every two persons would have had cancer in their lifetime. So, if you are married and have a child its likely one of you will encounter cancer. But the good news is, cancer is more lifestyle than it is genetic, and even genetic triggers can be turned off. So, with knowledge you can begin to increase the state of health of you and your family with some of the things I've talked about. But most importantly as a first response in conscious restoration by reducing sugar intake. Sugar is acidic, and the body is alkaline and so it creates an environment feeds cancer and other bacterial and inflammatory conditions which are often seen in people who get a serious ill health diagnosis like diabetes, hypertension, kidney failure, liver dis-ease or cancer.

Couple this with increasing your intake of wholefoods, water, sunlight and clean air and reducing exposure to radiation like cellphones, modems and other gadgets especially while sleeping can reduce your risk of cancer significantly. You can do it. It just takes discipline and a lot of could-care-less about what I've been taught, or what people think, to get there.

I always remind people that we have people in other continents living well over one hundred healthy and fully functional so why do we rob ourselves of thirty plus years. We only get one body vehicle on the earth so why don't we take the best care we can of it. And if it falls apart too early, we'll have to exit this side of life early as well.

We've been sold so much untruths that we embrace; things like women having a hysterectomy being happy, so they won't have any more periods, while there are eighty-year-old women in Africa and India still having babies (SMH). Lies never bring health so educate yourself enough for you and your family.

Thank you. *You've* left a legacy with me that I can leave with my children and relatives and friends. **You're** the best thing that has happened to me, although many won't believe it. Because of **You** I'll never be the same but only better.

I think many of us can't leave our children wealth and great material blessings, but we can give them knowledge on how to live healthy and take care of themselves and then they will be able to protect their resources and truly enjoy their lives. That is true health. It's a joy to see my kids enjoy a salad or the sunshine and water instead of sugared juice and even having them correct me sometimes about my lifestyle and eating activities. This is a legacy that will benefit generations long after I'm gone.

Lovingly Tan'Yah

Dear Cancer,

You have taught me so much especially that I can and need to keep learning. Even when my body physically couldn't go *You* showed me that my mind still could and then little by little it willed me to keep going. The desire to heal and recover my health fueled me. Now as I help others, I still keep learning even from them.

All dis-ease has the same foundation and the more severe ones are a progressive elaboration over time. So, to heal we must approach ourselves holistically as spiritual, mental, physical, emotional, social and even environmental beings with constant imbalances. We must engage these areas together although emphasis may be needed in the one or more areas that more urgently need help.

The human body is alkaline, mainly electrical and fluid, warm, filled with oxygen and so everything we take in through all those different parts must promote that balance. If it doesn't systems or parts of them begin to have challenges in functioning and the body has to respond. If it keeps up, we become exhausted from inside out and malfunction and shut down soon set in. It is that simple.

So, if you keep having a cold or sinus infection yet you still keep taking a high sugar diet with lots of cold foods like ice water and cold drinks you will remain damp inside and mucus will remain and eventual inflammation and infection will set in and then a dis-ease will be named.

All dis-eases no matter how severe can be healed but it will take very intense therapy and support for recovery to be realized by an individual. My father is almost eighty years old and is finally learning he must keep up with his recovery to maintain good health. Things he didn't do or like to do when he was young, he now must consistently do. Food he didn't like to eat he now has to and that's just the way it is. He even realizes that many of the things we need to do his grandmother did, so its nothing new. No wonder they lived real long back then. So, it's the old ways coming back to life through us to be given to the younger ones coming up. The mind is the most powerful tool in the healing process because it is the gateway to commitment. The mind must be willing to learn new pathways to health that were never taught.

Health and healing does come at a price. The cost is the stigma and ridicule you will face when you accept that doctors and conventional medicine don't know everything. As a global citizen you are entitled to information from other cultures so you can understand why there are over 500 cancer protocols globally that have proven some effectiveness in treating and even curing cancer in many cases. Health is no longer an individual, family, community or even national issue. To be a global citizen is to be able to access what I call 'Health Literacy'. Many of us are illiterate as to how to heal and stay healthy but it's not a lost cause because thanks to the world wide web, amazon books and many others sources like some of the elderly encyclopedia (old people) we have parked in senior homes, knowledge is out there and for the most part it's free so get to learning so you can get to living.

Resources I Used

- Cancer Tutor Website
- European medical journals
- Radical Remission – book and website
- Electromagnetic Energy treatments
- Detox treatments
- Coffee Enemas
- Ozone therapy
- Vitamin and herbal supplementation
- Conqueror support groups and mentors
- Emotional and spiritual restoration sessions
- Talk Therapy
- Creative arts mediums like creative visualization in writing or visual arts
- Laugh therapy like funny videos
- Traditional Chinese medicine sites and books
- Truth About Cancer Documentary Series
- Podcasts and online courses

This isn't all the things I did, but it is some of the most regularly used tools that I did use and still use today.

And I'm always learning ancient and new and emerging therapies to support healing and wellness. I'm still healing and growing in wellness.

Other Books

Created
Daughter
A 40 DAY
CHALLENGE
BY TAN'YA

A Compilation
LOVE
Never Fails
Tan'Ya Global

I am greater spiritually.
HEAVENLY EYES
byTan'Ya Global

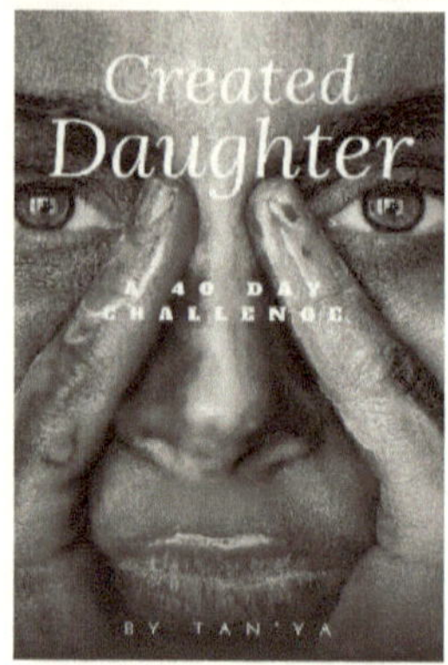

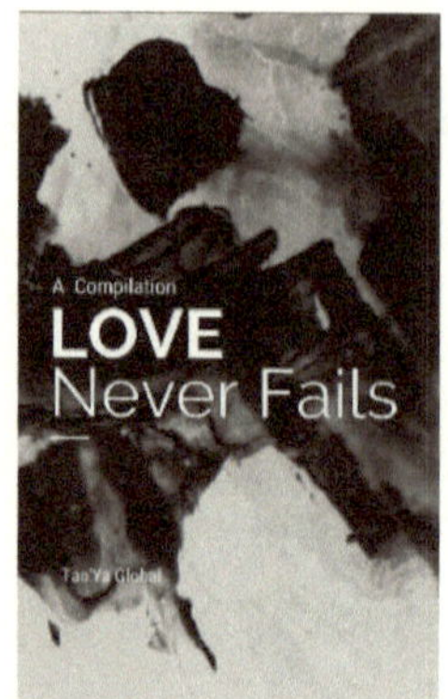

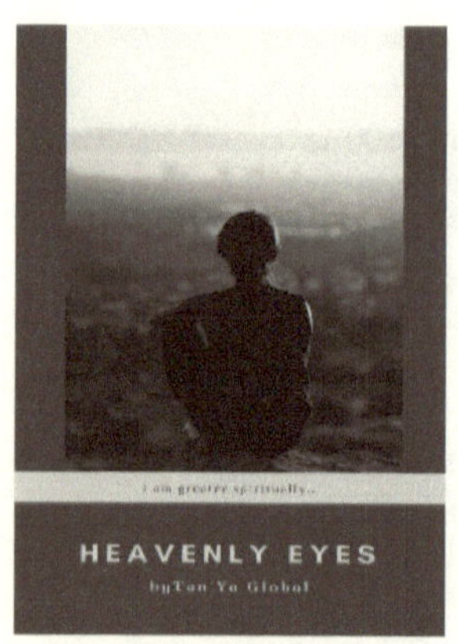

www.ingramcontent.com/pod-product-compliance
Lightning Source LLC
Chambersburg PA
CBHW051224250726

48655CB00006B/2582